32 WAYS TO OUTSMART CANCER

Create a body in which cancer cannot thrive.

DR. NALINI CHILKOV, L.AC., O.M.D.
FOUNDER, INTEGRATIVE CANCER ANSWERS

Do you really have the
power to outsmart cancer?

Yes!

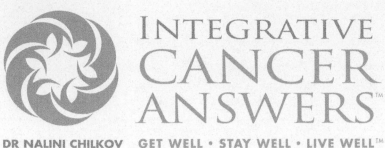

INTEGRATIVE
CANCER
ANSWERS™

DR NALINI CHILKOV   GET WELL • STAY WELL • LIVE WELL™

32 Ways to OutSmart Cancer:
Take Control of Your Health and Create A Body in Which
Cancer Cannot Thrive

by Dr. Nalini Chilkov, L.Ac., O.M.D.,
Founder, Integrative Cancer Answers

ISBN-13: 978-1500323462

DISCLAIMER

The information in this guide is not intended as medical or legal advice, or as a substitute for consultation with a physician or other licensed health care provider. Persons with health care related questions should call or see their physician or other health care provider promptly, and should not disregard professional medical advice, or delay seeking it, because of information encountered in this guide. The mention of any product, service, or treatment in this guide should not be construed as an endorsement. Integrative Cancer Answers is not responsible for any injury or damage to persons or property arising out of or related to any use of this guide, or to any errors or omissions.

ICA does not provide medical, diagnostic, or treatment advice. Information and statements regarding foods and dietary supplements have not been evaluated by the Food and Drug Administration and are not intended to diagnose, treat, cure, or prevent any disease.

DEDICATION

Dedicated to courageous hearts and spirits of my patients and their loved ones who have been my teachers. They have shown me what it means to open fully and tenderly to all of life.

It is my honor and privilege to be allowed to be part of such an intimate and profoundly transformational process of healing.

Praise for Dr. Nalini and Integrative Cancer Answers

Last year I almost died of advanced cancer. Nobody should have to go through what I experienced – My doctors are amazed. After only two weeks of starting my nutritional supplements, herbal medicines, morning smoothie and cancer fighting diet, my health and vitality doubled and in three months, I'm feeling close to 100%

– Dr. Nalini Chilkov is my secret weapon for perfect health – she's practical, pragmatic and brilliant.

Mike Koenigs
Advanced Colorectal Cancer
Best Selling Author and Speaker

Finally, someone who is looking at the whole and long term picture; not just deploying nuclear bombs in my body and waiting to see the results. Now I feel like I can be pro-active in my battle and not just a vessel for harmful but necessary chemicals. Some much of her nutritional advice, as my husband is a wonderful and informed cook, was on our radar but thanks to Dr. Chilkov, we now have the needed impetus to clean up those last nasty eating choices. Her encouragement to use this illness to create life changing habits was empowering and the comfort of knowing that she be in my corner for a long time to come is a huge emotional boost. Even the process of sorting through the plethora of vitamin/supplement bottles feels liberating and the acupuncture session was a definite boost to my energy level & well being. I cannot thank you enough for your all knowing kindness. With extreme gratitude for giving a life changing gift. I am not sure where to begin to thank you. My meeting with Dr. Chilkov was the most needed of medicines.

J.C., Cancer Patient

Her skill has helped me to heal physically. More importantly, her compassion and patience helped me to grow and develop as a human being. Rarely in life do you meet someone who wondrously heals and teaches. In so doing, they expand and change your life. Nalini is one of those rare people.

M.B., 21st Century Funds

You have treated me as a whole person, not just a list of ailments, and given me tools to add to the quality of my life in so many more ways than any doctor I have known. Thank you for helping me get well both physically, mentally and spiritually.

R.R., A.I.A.

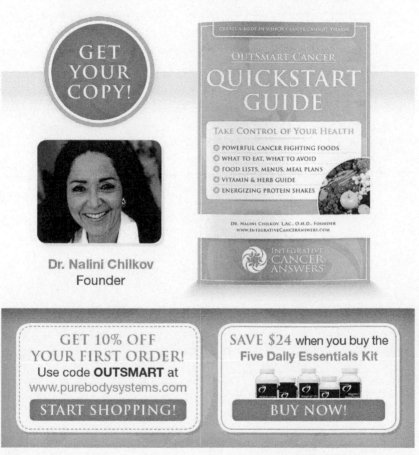

CONTENTS

INTRODUCTION

Let Me Take You on a Journey...

We now have the amazing opportunity to take the very best of modern science and combine it with ancient wisdom to nourish robust and lasting health and longevity. Let me take you on a journey and show you how to create and sustain real health, not just "the absence of symptoms." Let me show you what really matters and how to change your life.

As a Doctor Of Oriental Medicine, I apply the wisdom of an ancient system that understands the laws of nature. Oriental Medicine has continually grown and evolved with modern science and is now being used side-by-side in modern hospitals and medical settings in China, and even in some hospitals in America. Combined with 30 years of clinical experience caring for cancer patients, cancer survivors and those who do not want to get cancer in the first place in collaboration with physicians, I have distilled here the absolute essential steps you can take to create a body in which cancer cannot develop and thrive.

What Does it Really Mean to Take Control of Your Health and Your Destiny?

What does it really take to outsmart cancer, stop worrying, and enjoy real peace of mind? How can you arm yourself with reliable and trustworthy knowledge about your own health and future?

Your doctor is a disease expert, not a health expert. If you want to live a long disease-free life, you need to focus on health, not illness.

What will REALLY make a difference?

Cancer is about disease, illness, suffering, and "life and death." Cancer is quite possibly your biggest wake-up call and your greatest fear.

But what if cancer might actually be an empowering transformational healing journey, a gateway that changes you forever in ways you never imagined? Can you imagine saying: "Cancer is one of the best things that ever happened to me"? You would be surprised by how many people say this.

You don't want to be disease-free. You want to be healthy – robustly healthy – energized, joyous, and able to sleep at night because you are filled with deep peace in your heart and soul. And you want to dream, about a healthy future and long life.

Health is not just about surviving but about really thriving, living without anxiety and fear, and being filled with energy, vitality, and optimism.

Modern medicine is focused on disease, illness, and pathology. Let's walk away from disease and create health. I will show you how.

Sincerely,

Dr. Nalini Chilkov, L.Ac., O.M.D.

Cancer is Linked to the Way You Live and the Choices You Make

The Power to Live Robustly Well is in Your Hands

According to the National Institute of Health, 40% of all cancers can be prevented by simple lifestyle changes alone.

If people stopped smoking and overeating, limited their alcohol, exercised regularly and reduced exposures to toxic chemicals over the course of their lives, they would have a better chance of outsmarting cancer.

One of the most powerful choices you make every day is to choose what to eat. Simply by choosing the most powerful cancer-fighting superfoods, you will be on your way to outsmarting cancer naturally.

A Journey Begins With Just One Step...

This book contains 32 simple actions you can take right now to protect yourself, your children, your family, your loved ones.

Take just one action each week, and you will have transformed your risk and created an anti-cancer healthy life in only 8 months! Take two steps each week, and you can do it in 4 months. Take three steps each week and you will have changed your life in only 2 months! Wow, that is truly amazing.

Go at a pace that suits you. This is not a race. This is about intentionally creating the rest of your healthy, vibrant life!

Think long-term. One step at a time.

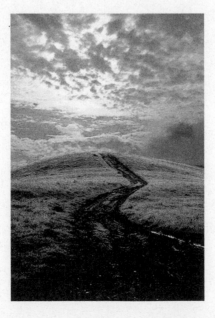

PART 1

Create an Anti-Cancer Body

CHAPTER 1

STOP SMOKING AND AVOID SECONDHAND SMOKE

Fact: Smoking causes cancer – cancer of the lungs, head, face, tongue, throat, nose and mouth. It isn't pretty and these cancers are VERY hard to treat. Not only does smoking cause cancer, but exposure to secondhand smoke causes cancer as well. So encourage any smokers around you to stop smoking.

Refuse to be in the presence of smoke.

This is a no-brainer, but if I failed to talk about it, that would just be irresponsible.

An addiction can be challenging to stop. Acupuncture is a very effective approach. I have seen some individuals stop smoking in less than a month.

Some people have a genetic trait that makes exposure to tobacco smoke dramatically more toxic and dangerous.

If you want to find out, ask your doctor to test you for **P450 enzyme CYP1B1 abnormalities.**

For your own life and the life of those around you, do whatever it takes to make your environment smoke-free.

If you smoke, make the decision to become a non-smoker.

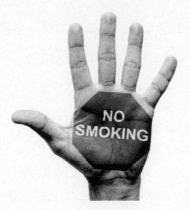

Chapter 2

Eat Anti-Inflammatory Foods, Herbs, and Spices

Food is information. Food "talks" to your DNA, telling it which genes to turn on and off. That's why it matters what you eat.

Follow an **anti-cancer anti-inflammatory diet** rich in cancer-fighting super foods, herbs, and spices. Choose foods that send healthy messages directly to your genes.

Remember, cancer is an inflammatory disease. Managing the cellular environment and modulating inflammation can reduce cancer-related symptoms and change a pro-cancer terrain to an anti-cancer terrain within your body. The ongoing presence of inflammation sets the stage for many diseases, including cancer. Lowering inflammation with plant chemicals found in common foods, herbs, and spices may contribute to turning off genes and inflammatory molecules that lead to the development, growth, and spread of cancer cells. Stop inflammation. Stop Cancer.

Simple steps for following an anti-inflammatory diet:

1. Include superfoods and spices that promote normal inflammatory control.

2. Eat more plant foods and less animal foods.

3. Introduce beans and legumes for some of your protein servings.

4. Consume more fresh fruits and vegetables (8-12 servings a day). Half of your plate should be vegetables at every meal (and no, ketchup is not a vegetable!). If you don't think you can do that, use a greens powder or a reds powder daily.

5. Eat lots of healthy fats and oils. A diet containing uncooked healthy fats and oils is an anti-inflammatory diet. Add high quality uncooked virgin olive oil in place of margarine, eat avocados and olives, almonds and walnuts. Don't fry your food.

6. Cook with herbs and spices that promote and enhance healthy levels of inflammation. Try adding turmeric, ginger root, oregano, thyme, basil and mint.

7. Eat something fermented every day: yoghurt, kefir, miso, natto, sauerkraut, or kim chi, for example.

8. Eliminate and avoid foods that trigger or promote increased levels of inflammation.

9. Read labels. Avoid processed, packaged foods containing:

   • Refined concentrated sugars

   • High fructose corn syrup

   • Chemical additives, preservatives, artificial colorings and flavorings, artificial sweeteners

10. Avoid grilled, charred blackened meats, fish, and poultry. Instead cook your meats by boiling, baking, steaming, roasting or cooking very slowly and lightly on the grill at a lower heat.

11. Reduce your intake of red meat to 1-2 servings weekly.

12. Avoid carbonated beverages, fried food, and trans fats (read labels).

13. Eliminate foods that trigger allergic reactions. The most common are cow's milk dairy products, gluten, gliadin-containing grains (wheat and wheat products, oats, barley and rye), eggs, soy, and peanuts.

14. Eat cancer-fighting superfoods such as deep green kale. It's rich in sulforaphanes, which support detoxification of environmental toxins and normal metabolism of estrogens that contribute to hormonal cancers such as breast and prostate cancer. Kale

is also uniquely high in the protective super antioxi-dant, lutein.

By choosing foods, herbs and spices that PROMOTE NORMAL INFLAMMATORY CONTROL and eliminating foods that ramp up inflammation in your cells and tissues, you can change the environment of your cells. Promote a physiology in which there are fewer triggers of inflammation and in which your own body is supported in normalizing inflammation. This is a very powerful step in creating an anti-cancer body.

Cancer – an Inflammatory Disease

Cancer is an inflammatory disease. **Inflammation*** is rampant among cancer patients and cancer survivors. Cancer-related fatigue, a distressing and persistent sense of physical and emotional tiredness, as well as reduced mental clarity and alertness may be linked to chronic persistent inflammation.

By taking steps to reduce **inflammation**, which is at the root of many cancers, you can begin your journey to an anti-cancer body and anti-cancer life.

* Learn More About 5 Natural Ways to Control Inflammation:

http://www.integrativecanceranswers.com/controlling-inflammation-five-natural-ways-to-put-out-the-fire/

CHAPTER 3

EAT A RAINBOW OF COLORS*
FROM FRESH ORGANIC
FRUITS AND VEGETABLES

To create an anti-cancer body, eat deeply and richly colored fruits and vegetables.

Nature is literally waving a brightly colored flag to get your attention. Many colorful plant pigments interact with your genes in a protective fashion. Each color in a fruit or vegetable gives you a gift directly from nature:

Red lycopene in tomatoes, red peppers, watermelon

Red quercetin in the skin of red apples and red onions

Orange carotenoids in carrots, winter squash, yams, mangos, cantaloupe

Green sulforaphanes in broccoli, kale, and lutein in spinach

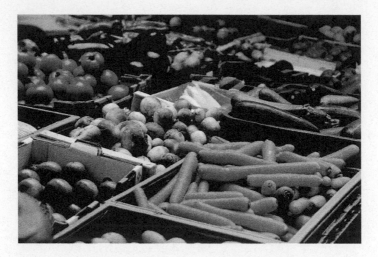

Blue-purple pterostilbene in blueberries

Red-purple resveratrol in red and purple grape and red wine

To get a good dose of cancer protection every day, aim for 8-12 servings of fruits and vegetables daily (1 serving = a cup or a handful) or simply be sure that HALF of your plate is vegetables at lunch and dinner!

* Learn More About How Colorful Fruits and Vegetables Fight Cancer:

http://www.integrativecanceranswers.com/cancer-fighting-foods-what-colors-are-on-your-plate/

CHAPTER 4

AT LEAST HALF OF YOUR FOOD SHOULD COME FROM PLANTS

Your food is talking to your genes, turning diseases on and off. It does matter what you eat!

A plant-based diet includes an emphasis upon fruits, vegetables, nuts, seeds, grains and beans. At every meal, half of your plate should be filled with vegetables.

Eating a plant-based diet immediately reduces your exposures to toxins and increases the amount of protective antioxidants that enter your body.

The many plant chemicals found in plant-based foods actually turn on cancer suppressor genes and turn off cancer promoter genes. Now that is amazing! Follow a diet that is at least 50% organic plant-based foods.

Plants are the primary source of cell protective **antioxidants** in the diet. The colors of fruits and vegetables show us the presence of these powerful messengers from nature, which are crucial to the protection your cells and your genes from damage that leads to cancer.

Plants are also your primary source of **fiber** necessary for normal intestinal function.

Choose Organic Whenever Possible

Vegetables grown in organic soil are known to contain more nutrients than commercially grown vegetables.

Whenever possible, choose organic produce that is in season. Eating food that is in season means it's fresh and full of nutrients.

Here are a few delicious vegetables you can try:

- Spinach, Swiss chard, kale, green leaf lettuce, red leaf lettuce

- Sweet potatoes, butternut squash, winter squash

- Zucchini, cucumbers, radishes, cauliflower, red bell peppers

- Broccoli, cabbage, Brussels sprouts, avocados

- Apples, peaches, strawberries, blueberries

- Blackberries, cantaloupe, honeydew, pomegranates

- Almonds, walnuts, sesame seeds, flax seeds, chia seeds

- Olives and olive oil

- Quinoa and buckwheat

- Lentils, black beans, chickpeas

The possibilities are endless. Mother nature provides an abundance of plants that supply nutrients to keep your body healthy.

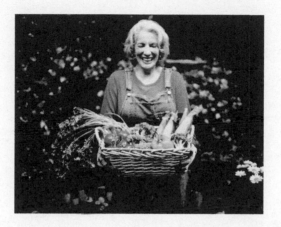

"This diagnosis is a reminder that this is the life you've got. And you're not getting another one. Whatever has happened, you have to take this life and treasure and protect it."

Elizabeth Edwards

"If you don't know your options, you don't have any."

Elyn Jacobs, breast cancer survivor

CHAPTER 5

DECREASE RED MEAT, ANIMAL FATS, AND ANIMAL PROTEINS

Decrease Your Exposure to Hormones in Food

To reduce exposures to hormones and environmental toxins concentrated in animal foods, decrease your consumption of red meat, animal fats and proteins.

All animal foods, flesh, and fats contain **hormones**. Humans eat primarily the meat, milk, and fat from the female animals. Growth hormones and estrogens are often added to animals feed to fatten them up.

Cancers promoted by hormonal stimulation can include breast, prostate, ovarian, uterine, lung, pancreatic, and colon cancer, to name a few. The environment is filled with chemicals that act like hormones such as **pesticides, herbicides and plastics.**

You can lower exposure to hormones in foods altogether by eating more, preferably organic, chemical free plant-based foods and less animal foods.

Decrease Your Exposure to Toxic Chemicals

The higher up on the food chain you eat, the more your food will be concentrated in environmental toxins.

Animal fats and proteins concentrate hormones and environmental chemicals.

Decrease Your Exposure to Excess Iron

Eating red meat is linked to increased rates of colon cancer. The high iron content found in red meat such as beef, lamb, and bison causes tissue damage because it is full of free radicals that pit your tissue just the way rust pits metal.

Remember that everything you eat touches the lining of your digestive organs and has a direct effect on your well-being!

Choose Wisely

When you do eat animal-based foods, such as eggs, dairy products, meat, milk, butter, and fish, remember to choose sources that are:

- Organic

- Free-range and Grass Fed

- Wild caught

- Free of hormones and antibiotics

- Free of artificial colorings and preservatives

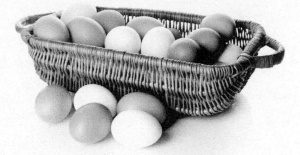

CHAPTER 6

KEEP INSULIN AND BLOOD SUGAR LOW BY AVOIDING SWEETS, SUGARS AND STARCHES

It is well-known that a diet low in sugars, starches, and sweets inhibits cancer growth.

Sugar is food for cancer cells. Starve cancer cells of sugar, and they become stressed and die.

A low glycemic diet (low in carbohydrates, sugars, sweets, fruits) is recommended for promoting not only an anti-cancer physiology but also an anti-diabetes, heart-healthy body. A diet high in sweets, starches and carbohydrates leads to both high blood sugar and high insulin, and a dramatic increase in cancer risk.

This topic is so important, I've written an entire book on it called *Sweets That Kill: The Link Between Sugar and Cancer*. High blood sugar, high blood insulin, pre diabetes, diabetes, being overweight and over fat are all linked to higher rates of cancer and cancer recurrence.

Let me say this again! High blood sugar, pre-diabetes, diabetes, and high insulin levels are linked to many cancers. Diabetics and pre-diabetics have an increased risk of cancer. One of the most powerful things you can do is **reduce your blood sugar, your blood insulin, and your body fat**. These steps alone have a dramatic impact on cancer rates. You can transform your metabolism by making changes in your food choices, your exercise, your sleep patterns and your sugar intake!

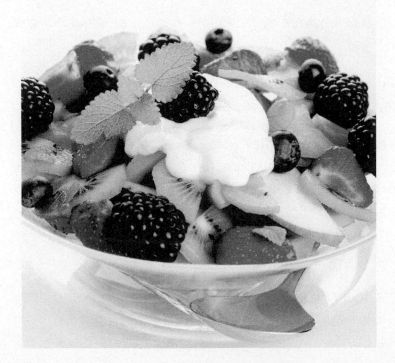

Recommended actions:

- Avoid all refined sugars and sweets

- Avoid concentrated fruit juices

- Limit fruit intake to 1-2 servings daily (emphasize vegetables instead)

- Eat a whole foods diet low in carbohydrates, low in sugar and sweeteners, low in starchy vegetables and grains and rich in healthy proteins, and healthy fats and green leafy vegetables

- Avoid all high fructose corn syrup

What does that look like?

Your plate should be half non-starchy green, yellow, and purple vegetables, 1/4 high quality protein, 1/8 healthy fats and oils, and 1/8 berries for dessert!

You may be able to change your physiology with changes in exercise, food choices, and stress management. Remember, food is information and is signaling your genes to promote health or promote disease, depending on what you eat. Send health promoting messages and you will have a healthier body!

My Outsmarting Cancer Naturally program devotes an entire module to making healthy food choices.

Available at www.IntegrativeCancerAnswers.com

CHAPTER 7

EAT HEALTHY FATS AND OILS DAILY

Including healthy fats and oils in your diet is one of the most powerful steps you can take to transform your health and create a body inhospitable to the growth of cancer.

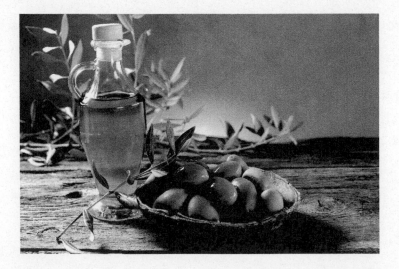

Healthy fats are a critical part of an anti-inflammatory diet.

Unfortunately, the modern diet is filled with **unhealthy fats** that contribute to unwanted inflammation.

Include healthy fats and oils at every meal, such as:

- olive oil

- flax seeds and flax oil

- walnuts and walnut oil

- avocados

- virgin coconut oil

- pine nuts

- wild-caught cold water fish such as salmon, cod, sardines, and mackerel

- high omega 3 eggs

- high omega 3 butter from grass-fed cows only

- high omega 3 meats from grass-fed animals (in small amounts only)

- Look for labels that say "no trans fat"

Avoid these fats and oils:

- Margarine and hydrogenated fats and oils

- Trans fats

- Lard, margarine, shortening

- Deep fried foods

- Rancid oils that are past the expiration date or which have not been properly stored

By eating MORE of these healthy fats, you will not only be following an anti-inflammation diet, you'll also be following a diet that is heart-healthy and anti-cancer.

CHAPTER 8

MAKE HIGH FIBER YOUR FRIEND

Increasing your fiber intake is one of many steps you can take to create an anti-cancer body.

A high fiber diet promotes normal healthy intestinal function, normal weight, and normal appetite control.

Plant fibers contribute to normal bowel function and support the growth of healthy bacteria in your gut – a key factor in robust immunity and estrogen excretion.

The fiber in whole foods is very important to regulating blood sugar.

Remember that plant foods are your main source of fiber:

- whole grains
- fruits

- vegetables
- nuts and seeds
- beans and legumes

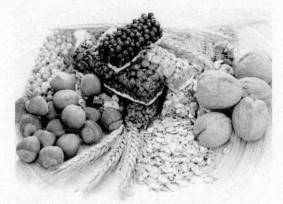

Not only are these plant-based foods your sources of fiber, but they are also rich sources of **phytochemicals** that act as super anti-oxidants. These have the capacity to turn on disease-fighting and cancer-fighting genes, as well as normalize inflammation and modulate immune function.

Start eating more fiber today. If you make a smoothie or shake for breakfast, try adding fiber powders, flax seed meal, or chia seeds for extra fiber.

CHAPTER 9

CREATE A "HEALTHY ECOLOGY" IN YOUR INTESTINES BY EATING FERMENTED FOODS

For a healthy digestive system and a robust immune system, make fermented foods a regular part of your diet.

Fermented foods such as yoghurt provide a nutritional dose of **friendly bacteria – including acidophilus.**

These beneficial bacteria are crucial for normal immunity, normal hormone clearance, normal inflammation control, as well as protection and repair of the digestive tract.

Without healthy bacteria, we would die. Having low levels or unhealthy types of bacteria can lead to serious illness, obesity and being overweight.

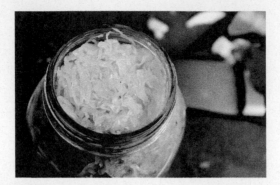

Make these foods a regular part of your diet:

- plain unsweetened yoghurt

- kefir

- coconut milk or almond milk products that are cultured with acidophilus

- miso, natto and tempeh (fermented soy products)

- fermented vegetable dishes (such as sauerkraut and kim chi made with cabbage, radishes and carrots)

Another way to get healthy friendly bacteria is to take a pill, capsule, or powder of a high-quality "probiotic" supplement usually made from acidophilus.

Fermented foods can help you nourish and maintain a normal immune system!

"Getting cancer can become the beginning of
living. The search for one's own being,
the discovery of the life one needs to live, can be
one of the strongest weapons against disease."

Lawrence Leshan

CHAPTER 10

FEAST ON CABBAGE FAMILY VEGETABLES* AND GARLIC

All of the cabbage family vegetables contain compounds called **sulforaphanes**, which promote detoxification function and modulate hormones.

Cabbage family vegetables include:

- broccoli
- kale
- cauliflower
- Brussels sprouts
- radishes

Sulforaphanes:

- Promote detoxification of environmental chemicals, hormones and toxins

- Promote normal inflammation control

- Support protective antioxidant functions reducing damage

Sulphoraphanes found in cabbage family vegetables may be linked to reduced risk of many cancers such lung, stomach, colorectal, prostate, cervical and bladder cancers.

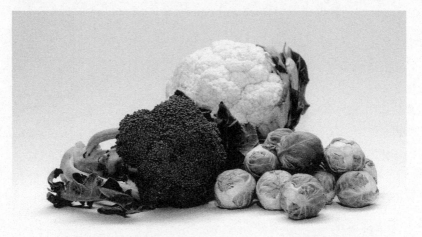

The Importance of Sulfur-Rich Foods

All of the cabbage family vegetables and all of the onion and garlic family vegetables contain **high amounts of sulfur**, known for its detoxifying properties.

Garlic, rich in sulfur, is particularly valuable because it not only promotes detoxification functions, but also supports normal immune resistance to infections from bacteria and viruses.

Garlic also provides pre-biotic fibers that promote the growth of healthy friendly bacteria in the digestive tract, so crucial to normal immunity.

Garlic can be added to soups, vegetables dishes, sauces and dressings, or taken in capsule form. It can be eaten raw, chopped up into little pieces and swallowed like pills.

For a boost of cancer-fighting compounds, include cabbage family vegetables and garlic in your diet on a regular basis.

* Learn More About the Five Benefits of Eating Broccoli:

http://www.integrativecanceranswers.com/your-mom-was-right-5-reasons-to-eat-your-broccoli/

CHAPTER 11

PROTECT YOUR GENES BY COOKING WITH SPICES AND HERBS RICH IN ANTICANCER PLANT CHEMICALS

Cook with pungent and flavorful spices and herbs rich in anti-cancer phytochemicals that promote normal inflammatory function and protect your DNA.

Try these amazing herbs and spices:

- **Turmeric** (the source of curcumin) is one of the most potent anti-cancer spices in your kitchen

- Bright red **Paprika** contributes anti-cancer carotenoid lycopene.

- **Ginger root** supports normal inflammation function and enhanced digestive function

- **Rosemary** is rich in carnosol, cell protective compound

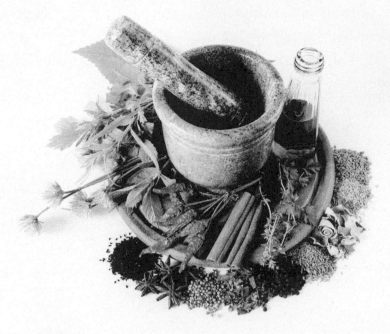

- **Thyme** is rich in essential oils that support digestion and protect cells

- **Mints** contain oils that enhance normal intestinal function

- **Parsley** contains apigenin important in normal cell function

- **Oregano** contains compounds that promote healthy cell function

- **Basil** contributes phytochemicals that support normal cell signaling

- **Saffron** is rich in protective carotenoids

- **Garlic** is rich in sulfur and allicilin which support normal detoxification function

Not only do these herbs and spices offer protective cancer-fighting properties, they also enhance digestive function and infuse your food with aroma and delicious flavors.

CHAPTER 12

AIM FOR 3 SERVINGS OF CLEAN, HIGH-QUALITY PROTEIN DAILY

Eat protein at every meal to support stamina, endurance, and immunity.

Protein is required to build the army of your immune system, including infection-fighting antibodies and cancer-fighting "Natural Killer Cells." Proteins help with repair, while keeping the barriers to infection (the linings of your nose, throat, lungs, digestive tract, and skin) intact.

Protein is essential to the brain and to the health of every cell.

Eat 20 grams or 4 ounces (which is about a handful of protein) 3 times daily.

* Consult with your doctor about how much and what kind of protein is right for you.

Protein is available from many sources, including:

- **Whey protein.** Choose high-quality whey that is non-heat treated and undenatured. Whey is one of the highest quality proteins. It is made from a highly purified fraction of milk. Some people with dairy sensitivities or allergies should be careful with whey protein.

- **Rice or pea or hemp protein powder.** You can mix this into a shake with berries and coconut milk for a delicious, well-balanced meal.

- **Grass-fed meat.** Always choose free range, organic, grass-fed, hormone-free, antibiotic-free sustainable meat products.

- **Poultry (chicken, turkey).** Choose the best-quality poultry from free-range animals raised without hormones, antibiotics, or pesticides

- **Wild caught, coldwater ish.** Wild Alaskan salmon is an excellent source of protein. Avoid large fish such as swordfish, tuna, and tilefish, which are often high in mercury and other contaminants. Consult www.seafoodwatch.com to choose the safest fish all year round.

- **Eggs.** Choose high omega 3, organic, hormone-free eggs.

- **Dairy Products** such as cheese, cottage cheese, milk, whey, yoghurt and kefir. The casein and lactose found in dairy products can trigger food sensitivities

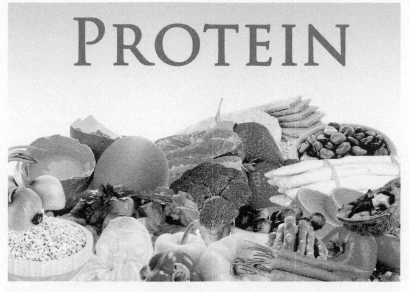

and allergic and inflammatory reactions. Check with your doctor before adding any new food to your diet.

A great strategy for getting enough high-quality protein is to make a protein shake or smoothie for breakfast every day.

Instead of eating toast, fruit, pancakes, oatmeal, cereal, or potatoes and other high-carbohydrate foods, emphasize protein for breakfast. You'll have high energy throughout the day. And you won't be eating a meal that looks like dessert for breakfast!

Choose leftover dinner such as soup, fish or chicken and vegetables for breakfast. Try organic chicken or turkey sausages, cottage cheese, Greek yoghurt, almonds, almond butter, tofu or beans and yes...vegetables for breakfast!!

CHAPTER 13

DRINK GREEN TEA REGULARLY

To protect your body against free radicals and increase protection to your genes, drink green tea daily.

One of the most widely studied plants, green tea is a "multi-tasker." It has many protective functions. The beauty of plant medicine is that there are many gifts from just one plant!

The science behind green tea is compelling:

- Green tea is the source of potent **antioxidant** plant **polyphenols**, including cell protectant Epigallocatechin gallate (ECGC).

- ECGC has demonstrated anti-tumor activity as well as modulation of fatigue, mental clarity, thinking, and memory.

- **ECGC** has been shown to decrease levels of inflammatory molecules linked to the development of can-

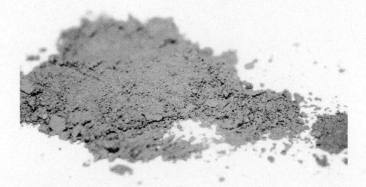

cer and many chronic diseases (TNFa, IL-1B and NFkB.) Decreasing inflammation is a key to creating a body inhospitable to cancer.

• **Green tea polyphenols** have also been shown to normalize fat metabolism.

To create an anti-cancer body, consider drinking 1-4 cups of green tea daily. Green tea does contain caffeine and tannins. If you are sensitive to either, check with your doctor before adding green tea to your diet.

"Pain is a part of life ... but suffering is optional."

Cancer Survivor

Chapter 14

Limit Alcohol Intake to Reduce Cancer Risk

More Alcohol More Cancer: The Numbers Tell a Grim Story

Reducing Alcohol saves lives.

Regular alcohol intake, just two drinks per day is linked to increased risk of many cancers, including breast cancer.

Women who drink two or more drinks daily have a 20% overall higher risk of dying of cancer. For every additional drink you have per day your risk goes up another 10%. Three drinks = 30% higher risk. Four drinks = 40% higher risk.

Just three drinks per week is linked to 15% increased risk of breast cancer, especially estrogen hormone sensitive cancers.

These levels of alcohol consumption are associated not only with a greater risk of cancer development but also a greater risk of cancer progression and cancer recurrence.

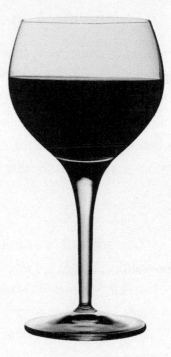

What to do? The key is MODERATION.

Limit your alcohol intake to 4 ounces per day. Even better, don't drink daily. Drink occasionally.

With red wine you get the benefit of cell protective resveratrol, a plant antioxidant found in the skin of red grapes. Resveratrol is one of the only plant chemicals with research to demonstrate that it actually protects your DNA from damage and thus pro-motes longevity!

Remember that alcohol is a sugar and does raise your blood sugar and trigger the release of insulin, both of which promote a biological environment that may promote cancer. One of the principles of an ant-cancer diet is a low glycemic diet" meaning a diet that is low in sugars, sweets, carbohydrates and starches.

Healthy Non-Alcoholic Choices

Instead of wine drink still or sparkling water with a splash of pomegranate, dark cherry or cranberry juice and little lemon or lime. Or make ice cubes out of these ruby colored juices and add them to your water glass. Or add a few organic strawberries or raspberries to your glass with a sprig of fresh mint or basil!

"Consult not your fears but your hopes and your dreams. Think not about your frustrations, but about your unfulfilled potential. Concern yourself not with what you tried and failed in, but with what is still possible for you to do."

Pope John XXIII

CHAPTER 15

KEEP YOUR BODY WEIGHT NORMAL

Keep your weight and body fat at a healthy level, and you may reduce your risk of getting cancer.

Researchers have discovered that as body fat increases, so do the rates of breast cancer, recurrence, and death.

According to The Breast Cancer Prevention and Treatment Fund, 20-30% of the most common cancers in the United States "may be related to being overweight and/or lack of physical activity."

In fact, **obesity** may become the biggest cause of cancer. Why? Because fat cells are "factories" for hormones and inflammation, both of which fuel the growth, development, and spread of breast cancer.

Research has shown that ovarian, endometrial, colorectal, prostate, pancreatic, and breast cancers are linked to excess body fat.

Here are some facts to consider:

- Body Fat makes **estrogen**, which fuels hormone-driven breast cancers.

- Fat tissue produces **inflammation**, which increases the development, growth, and spread of cancer, as well as many other chronic conditions.

- Fat tissue sends signals to the immune system, leading to **decreased immune response.**

- Fat tissue leads to changes in the function of insulin, an important hormone that regulates blood sugar. Extra body fat may promote dangerous **elevation in blood sugar,** obeslty, pre-diabetes, and diabetes – all of which increase your risk of breast cancer.

- Furthermore, **insulin** plays a role in tumor growth.

- The higher the insulin blood levels in breast cancer patients, the **greater the chance of death.**

- Excess body fat is the most dangerous for women with hormonal breast cancers, tumors with receptors for estrogen and progesterone (female hormones) and androgens (male hormones).

- Being overweight and having excess body fat puts you at risk for developing cancer, having a **cancer recurrence** and a lower chance of survival.

- One of the most powerful things you can do to lower cancer risk is to achieve a normal body weight, lose fat, and build muscle.

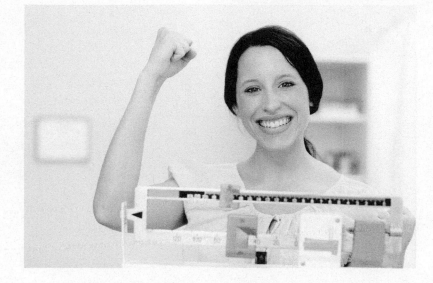

You can reduce your body fat by eating foods that promote fat metabolism (e.g., dark leafy green vegetables, cruciferous vegetables, and green tea), reducing your sugar intake, and incorporating regular aerobic and muscle-building exercise into your daily life.

CHAPTER 16

EXERCISE FOR AT LEAST 30 MINUTES FIVE DAYS PER WEEK AND SWEAT REGULARLY

To shift into an anti-cancer, pro-health physiology, you should do a minimum of 30 minutes of moderate exercise five days a week (or a total of 150 minutes per week), plus two days of strength training.

Check with your doctor first!

Moderate exercise can impact cancer risk by helping you:

1. Maintain a healthy weight. Increased body fat increases your risk of cancer.* Body fat acts as a factory for producing inflammation and hormones that contribute to a pro-cancer physiology. Overweight and obese individuals have increased rates of cancer and cancer recurrence. This may be your biggest risk factor.

2. Maintain normal blood sugar* metabolism and normal insulin signaling and reducing the risk of diabetes. Elevated blood sugar, diabetes, and pre-diabetes, also known as insulin resistance or metabolic syndrome, can fuel cancer growth. Diabetics with chronically elevated blood sugar, insulin and Insulin Like Growth Factor (IGF-1) levels have increased risk of cancer and cancer progression. Why? **Cancer cells preferentially utilize sugar as a fuel.**

The more sugary your blood, the more ready fuel is available for cancer cell growth. Elevated insulin and IGF-1 levels also promote cancer cell growth. Exercise not only **reduces body fat*** and increases muscle mass, but also influences hormone signaling to normalize blood sugar metabolism. The key is here is MODERATE exercise. Very intense exercise can trigger the release of cortisol, a hormone that elevates blood sugar.

3. Maintain healthy bones and muscles. Maintaining muscle mass is crucial to cancer survival. The loss of muscle mass is a risk factor for cancer progression. By maintaining healthy bones, there is less bone loss and fewer fractures. Healthy bone is also more resistant to invasion by cancer cells and the spread of cancer to the bone (bone metastases).

4. Maintain a robust immune system. Research supports the link between regular moderate exercise and a strong immune system. Physical activity promotes **production of immune cells**, including Natural Killer

Cells, which target both tumor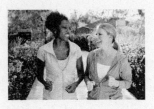
cells and viral cells. Some can-
cers are linked to viral infections.
For example, both cervical cancer
and head and neck cancers of the
mouth and throat are linked to Human Papilloma Virus
(HPV).

*Warning: Moderate exercise can boost immune system
function, but intense exercise can have the opposite
effect.*

5. Maintain healthy hormone levels. Exercise may
lower cancer risk by lowering insulin and insulin-like
growth factors, which are both cancer-promoting hormones. Increased body fat is coupled with increased
estrogen production from fat cells. Estrogen is related
to breast, uterine, and prostate cancers. By maintaining
normal weight and body fat, the risk of increased estrogen levels is reduced.

6. Maintain healthy mood and emotions. Exercise
has both psychological and biological effects on mood,
including feelings of depression, anxiety, and fatigue.
This of course impacts quality of life.

7. Maintain a strategy of stress management. Exercise can reduce psychological stress and tension, but
exercise also has a biological impact on stress. Because
ongoing stress may diminish the strength of the immune
system, moderate exercise supports a normal immune

system that more readily recognizes and destroys cancer cells.

8. Maintain an anti-cancer, health-promoting lifestyle.

- Cancer patients who exercise regularly are able to complete their treatments and suffer from fewer side effects compared to patients who are sedentary.

- Cancer patients who exercise have overall better rates of survival and lower rates of recurrence.

- Cancer survivors who maintain an active lifestyle have lower rates of new cancers.

- Cancer patients who exercise regularly have lower levels of biological markers related to cancer growth and progression.

- Cancer survivors who exercise are "Cancer Thrivers" and report increased quality of life.

Remember, REGULAR MODERATE EXERCISE AND ACTIVITY = LESS CANCER RISK, less stress, increased weight loss, better sleep, improved mood, less risk of heart disease, and a better quality of life.

Exercise transforms cancer risk and enhances immune robustness. A lifetime of regular exercise has the most benefit, but it is never too late to start! So get out your walking shoes, do some gardening, go for a bike ride, climb stairs, do some yoga or tai chi, and smell the roses.

* 1. Learn More About How Increased Body Fat Increases Your Risk of Cancer:

http://www.integrativecanceranswers.com/leading-cause-of-breast-cancer-overweight-women-at-highest-risk/

* 2. Learn More About The Dangers of Sugars and Starches:

http://www.integrativecanceranswers.com/breast-cancer-after-menopause-beware-of-sugars-and-starches/cancer

* 3. Learn More About How to Burn Fat:

http://www.peertrainer.com/diet/how-do-you-burn-fat.aspx

CHAPTER 17

STAY FIT AND LEAN WITH CARDIOVASCULAR EXERCISE, HIGH INTENSITY INTERVAL TRAINING, AND MUSCLE BUILDING

Maintaining muscle is crucial to cancer survival. The loss of muscle mass is linked to fatigue, weakness, lowered resistance, cancer progression and even death.

Exercise also promotes bone health. By maintaining healthy bones, there is less bone loss and fewer fractures. Healthy bone is also more resistant to invasion by cancer cells and the spread of cancer to the bone (bone metastases).

Weight training, strength training, and muscle building are excellent ways to strengthen bones. The actual work of holding up your skeleton and your muscles pulling on bones keeps your bones strong.

Consider activities such as:

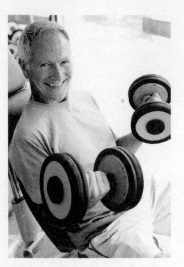

- yoga or tai chi

- weight lifting

- kettle balls

- muscle-strengthening exercises with weights or machines

- gardening, hiking, bike-riding, brisk walking

- dancing

Engage in regular aerobic cardiovascular and high-intensity interval training as well as muscle strengthening and muscle building exercises. Stay fit. Stay lean. Start with 10 minutes a day. Then build up little-by-little until you can do 30 minutes.

Check with your doctor before starting or changing your exercise routine.

CHAPTER 18

USE SUN PROTECTION

If you are fair-skinned, you should take extra measures to protect your skin from the sun.

It is widely known that sun exposure can cause skin cancer, including serious life threatening melanoma. However, not everyone who spends a lot of time in the sun gets skin cancer.

A fair-skinned individual may always get a sunburn, while another person gets a dark bronze tan and rarely burns. This is due to genetics.

The person who gets the golden brown tan has **genetic programming** that leads to the efficient production of melanin, the skin pigment that blocks the sun. **Melanin** acts as the body's natural sunscreen and also as an antioxidant in the skin. But don't be fooled excess sun exposure is risky even if you have dark skin.

It is known that early humans who roamed outside all day long near the equator had darker skin, a smart evolutionary trait to protect them from the effects of sun exposure. Over time, as humans wandered the earth and migrated to northern latitudes, they wore skins and furs to protect them from the cold. Farther from the equator, humans had less need for melanin-rich dark skin.

If your ancestors come from northern latitudes, they may have fair skin and be at higher risk for skin cancer, because they've lost the skin's natural ability to protect itself from the sun by producing dark pigmentation.

To protect yourself from sun damage, follow these tips:

- Get some **sun exposure on your skin without sunscreen** for 20-30 minutes in the morning or late afternoon – to ensure you produce adequate **Vita-**

min D. Use sunscreen during the midday to protect your skin.

• Avoid direct sunlight between 10 a.m. and 4 p.m. (peak burning hours)

• If you're in the sun during midday, wear a hat and cover yourself up with loose, long-sleeved shirts.

• Use an organic sunscreen that is free of toxic chemicals, with an SPF15 or higher.

• Avoid using tanning booths and sun lamps.

Remember, too much exposure to the sun at peak hours can lead to skin cancer. By protecting your skin, you may avoid skin cancer and stay looking younger longer.

Chapter 19

Get 7-9 Hours of Sleep*
Every Night

To avoid setting the stage for cancer, aim for 7-9 hours of high-quality sleep each night.

Getting sufficient sleep allows your immune system to increase the production of **"Natural Killer Cells"** that specialize in destroying both cancer cells and viral infections.

Adequate sleep is a contributor to normal immune function and crucial to cancer control.

Plentiful, high-quality sleep gives you a nightly dose of the brain hormone and super antioxidant, **melatonin**.

Breast cancer has been linked to the hormone melatonin, which regulates your sleep-wake cycle. Fluctuations in normal nighttime production of melatonin may be a predictor of whether or not you might develop breast cancer.

Here are 5 tips for getting a good night's sleep:

- **Relax and unwind in the hours before bedtime.** Create a nightly ritual in which you prepare yourself for sleep and help you wind down after a busy day. Turn off the computer and TV. Try gentle stretching, meditation, taking a hot bath, or enjoying a relaxing cup of caffeine-free herbal tea such as chamomile. Lavender oil has also been used traditionally in a relaxing bath or for scenting the pillow to promote relaxation.

- **Put yourself to bed earlier.** Human beings are keyed into the rhythm of nature and the cycles of dark and light. You must sleep when it is dark and wake when it is light to have normal physiology, including normal production of melatonin. When you start to feel sleepy, melatonin is being secreted, getting you ready for sleep. Heed the call.

- **Aim for 8 hours of good quality sleep.** Most people need 7-9 hours of sleep each night, which is when deep sleep occurs. It is during deep sleep that your body resets, re-patterns, restores, and heals.

- **Sleep in a truly dark room.** Even small amounts of light from LEDs from clocks and other electronic devices should be turned off or covered so that the room can be as completely dark as possible. Darkness signals the brain to produce melatonin.

- **Check your melatonin levels.** See your health care provider to measure your melatonin levels. If you are low, you may consider supplementing with 1-3 mg of melatonin at bedtime. Although melatonin is available over the counter, you should always consult with your doctor before taking any supplement.

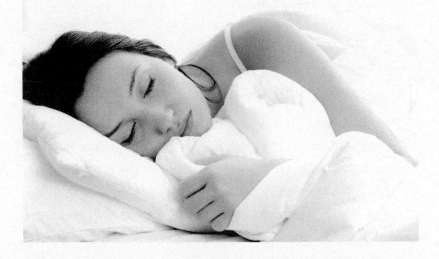

You can gradually retrain your body to fall asleep, stay asleep, and wake up refreshed and rested – so you can give your cells the opportunity to be exposed to melatonin, while putting cancer cells to sleep as well.

* Learn More About The Link Between Lack of Sleep and Cancer:

http://www.integrativecanceranswers.com/is-breast-cancer-linked-to-lack-of-sleep/

Chapter 20

Relax, Manage Stress*, and Take Sacred Time for Yourself

A few minutes of simply resting and breathing deeply can be extraordinarily restorative. By resting in tranquility and equipoise even for just 5 or 10 minutes, you begin to re-pattern your nervous system, your immune system, and your stress response. In doing so, your Natural Killer Cells – the cells in your immune system that fight cancer and infections – increase.

When you de-stress, several things happen:

- Stress hormones such as cortisol decrease

- Your heart rate slows

- Your breathing deepens

- Your muscles relax

- And even better....a little peace of mind just might save your life

Stress of all types damages the immune system and makes you more vulnerable to infections and cancer (and depression).

Stress depletes B vitamins, C, magnesium and zinc. You can eat nuts, seeds, berries, and fermented foods to replenish these deficiencies.

The best thing to do is relax. Get a massage. Watch the sunset. Gaze at the moon. Sink into a hot bath. Take a deep breath. Stop for just a few minutes and restore yourself. The benefits to your immune system will be immense.

* Learn 16 Tips for Managing Stress:

http://www.integrativecanceranswers.com/16-tips-for-managing-stress-preventing-burnout/

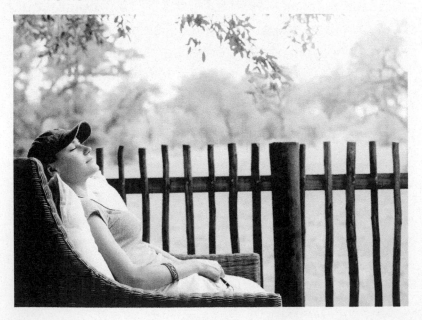

CHAPTER 21

ADD YOGA, TAI CHI, MEDITATION*, PRAYER, ACUPUNCTURE, AND MASSAGE INTO YOUR LIFE

Research has shown that complementary treatments (or "integrative therapies," as I like to call them) can effectively reduce stress if they are followed consistently over a long period of time.

Treatments and practices such as yoga, tai chi, Reiki, meditation, prayer, therapeutic massage, and acupuncture can all help you center yourself while relieving stress.

It's important to remember that **stress damages your immune system** and makes you more vulnerable to cancer. Cancer is stressful every step of the way, from diagnosis, through treatment and as a survivor worried about recurrence.

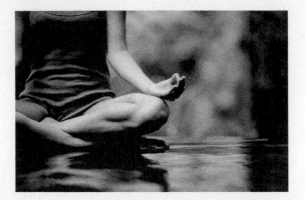

Actions that involve slow, deep breathing – and simply "slowing down" everything – can calm the nervous system, relieving you of stress.

Try following a daily or weekly de-stressing ritual to remind you to slow down and give yourself a rest. Which complementary treatment you choose may be somewhat less important than the fact that you choose one or more and follow through. In other words: **find something you like and stick with it.**

* Learn More About The Benefits of Meditation for Cancer Patients:

http://www.integrativecanceranswers.com/meditation-for-cancer-patients-and-the-rest-of-us/

PART 2

Take Control of Environmental Factors

CHAPTER 22

AVOID CHEMICAL EXPOSURES AT HOME AND WORK

Chemical exposures are a fact of modern life. As part of your journey to creating an anti-cancer body, begin to build awareness of the many sources of toxins in our daily lives, and take steps to make your home and work environments safe for you and your family.

It is pretty shocking to discover how many chemicals you are exposed to in your everyday environment and the toxic substances that you actually put into and on your body.

Substances such as **pthalates, parabens, chemical dyes and colorings, pesticides and herbicides** really don't belong on your skin or in your stomach. Nonetheless, they are found in many personal body care products and cosmetics, as well as in certain foods and common household cleaning supplies.

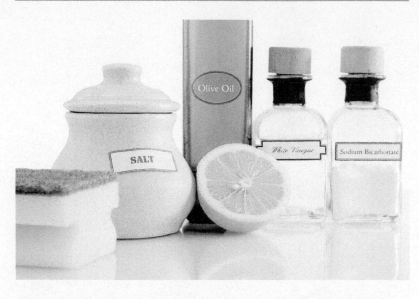

A recent study in the journal Environmental Health Perspectives points out that the state of product labeling in the U.S. is pretty poor. How poor? The study's researchers – who analyzed samples from 213 different consumer products ranging from cat litter to shaving cream, sunscreen, dishwater detergent, mascara, and vinegar – detected some 55 toxic chemicals. Many of these, they report, weren't listed on the labels of products tested.

It is important to read labels even on so-called "healthy" products. For example, there are more cancer-causing toxic chemicals in your shampoo than meets the eye.

It's best to select **non-toxic** shampoos, lotions, soaps, detergents, paints, and floor cleaners, and get a good water filter for your home.

Go through each room in your house one at a time. Discard anything with chemicals known to be harmful.

Avoid:

- parabens, pthalates, and Bisphenol A (BPA)
- artificial colorings, flavorings, and preservatives
- chemical dyes, artificial scents and fragrances
- aluminum
- Styrofoam

A great resource is www.everydayexposures.com, which can help you learn about the many toxins in your home, garden, and garage so you can make safer choices.

"The PART can never be well unless
the WHOLE is well."

Plato

CHAPTER 23

REMOVE CANCER-CAUSING PRODUCTS FROM YOUR HOME

Go through each room in your house and remove cancer-causing chemicals, cleaners, and body care products.

Every day, you use a myriad of personal care products on your body from soaps and lotions to shampoos and conditioners, makeup, and shaving creams. The ingredients in personal care products are largely unregulated. Chemicals found in cosmetics and personal care products are currently unregulated. Ingredients such as **pthalates, coal tar, talc and parabens** have been linked to increased risk of cancer. Many have been banned in Europe but not in the United States.

You may not know the extent to which you're exposed to environmental chemicals right in your own home. You can't eliminate all risk or exposure, but you can make significant changes to protect yourself and your family.

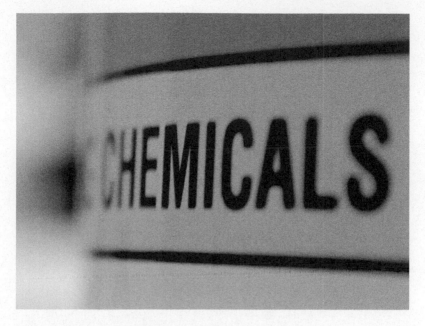

Here are a few tips to purify your home:

- Fill your home with plants to detoxify the air.

- Use HEPA filters and ionizers to reduce dust, molds, and off-gassing and fumes from synthetic carpets, furniture, and paints.

- Clean your heating systems and monitor them for carbon monoxide.

- Replace your cleaning supplies with non-toxic household products.

- Substitute fluorescent lights with incandescent or LED bulbs wherever possible.

- Filter your tap water with a simple carbon filter or a reverse-osmosis filtering system, then carry it with you in BPA-free stainless steel or glass bottles. (BPA is one of the most ubiquitous and toxic chemicals in our modern environment. It is used to make plastic found in food and drink containers.)

• If you use cosmetics, check EWG's Skin Deep Cosmetics Database (www.ewg.org/skindeep) to find out how toxic your products are.

• Minimize your exposure to electronic pollution. Mitigate any potential risks of electromagnetic radiation or electromagnetic frequencies by using an air tube headset or speakerphone **when talking on your cell phone*** (wireless and wired may still conduct radiation); keeping your smart phone at least 6-7 inches away from your body whenever in use; replacing as many cordless and WiFi items as you can with wired, corded lines; and sitting as far back from the computer screen as possible.

To reduce your risk of cancer due to exposure to chemicals, replace all toxic products with green, safe, non-toxic cosmetic and cleaning products for kitchen, laundry, and bath.

* Learn More About the Health Risks of Cell Phone Use:

http://www.integrativecanceranswers.com/health-risks-of-cell-phone-use/

CHAPTER 24

EAT WHOLE, UNPROCESSED ORGANIC FOODS

Eating organic foods is by far one of the most important things you can do to reduce your exposure to toxic chemicals, herbicides, pesticides, antibiotics, colorings and waxes – all of which have negative impact on health, immunity, and brain function, while increasing the risk of diseases such as multiple sclerosis and many cancers.

Organic foods are free of these toxic chemicals, as well as additives, artificial flavorings, steroids, and hormones.

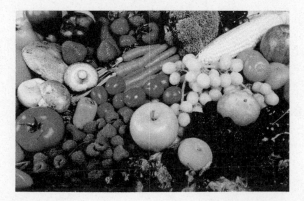

When eating organic is not possible due to budgetary constraints, seasonal unavailability, or lack of access to local farmer's markets, remember "The Dirty Dozen" and "The Clean 15." (from www.ewg.org)

The "Dirty Dozen" are 14 soft-skinned **foods that absorb the most pesticides** and which you must always buy organic.

They include:

1. Celery
2. Peaches
3. Strawberries
4. Apples
5. Domestic blueberries
6. Nectarines
7. Sweet bell peppers
8. Spinach
9. Kale
10. Collard Greens
11. Cherries
12. Potatoes
13. Imported Grapes
14. Lettuce

The "Clean 15" are foods that contain little to no pesticides, due to their strong outer layer that provides a defense against pesticide contamination. You can safely eat these foods even if they are not organic.

These include:

1. Onions

2. Avocados

3. Sweet corn

4. Pineapples

5. Mango

6. Sweet peas

7. Asparagus

8. Kiwi fruit

9. Cabbage

10. Eggplant

11. Cantaloupe

12. Watermelon

13. Grapefruit

14. Sweet potatoes

15. Sweet onions

Whenever possible, always choose organic – or at the very least, buy "The Dirty Dozen" in organic to ensure you're not ingesting high amounts of pesticides.

There is no doubt in my mind that reducing exposure to toxic chemicals – including pesticides – is important for long-term health.

Quick Tip: See the "Doctor-Nutritionist Designed Organic Frozen Meals" section at the end of this document for information on how to order healthy, delicious organic meals made by Artisan Bistro Pro. They are shipped right to your door.

"May we appreciate this divine place. May each one of us find details to caress. May we love this life, just as it is."

Insight Meditation Society Prayer

CHAPTER 25

DO A CLEANSE TO DETOXIFY YOUR BODY AT LEAST TWICE A YEAR

Detoxify your body of chemical load at least twice each year in spring and fall under the guidance of a knowledgeable health care professional.

A "detox" (also known as a cleanse) involves adding nourishing nutrients to your diet, while removing all chemicals, sugars, caffeine and inflammation-causing foods like gluten, dairy, soy, corn, eggs, peanuts, sugar, and alcohol.

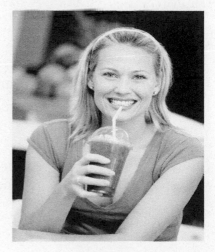

Detoxing is a great way to "reset" your body and return back to health. When done correctly, a detox should be restorative and nourishing, while supporting healthy bodily function.

Once you experience the extraordinary clarity, increased energy, and an increased sense of well-being you will make a decision to avoid chemical exposures in the first place whenever possible.

To start, try removing ALL of the following foods from your diet for 1 week:

- sugar, sodas, and artificial sweeteners
- wheat and wheat products
- soy, dairy, corn, eggs, peanuts
- all grains
- caffeine and alcohol
- packaged foods

For best results, consult a qualified health professional before embarking upon a cleanse or making changes to your diet.

For a balanced approach to whole body detox, explore the **Pure Body Cleanse**, designed to gently support cancer patients, survivors, thrivers – and anyone wishing to avoid cancer in the future or in the future.

For more information: **www.PureBodySystems.com**

Our Gift To You.

Get **10% Off Your First Order** for

Superior Professional Grade Supplements at our

Pure Body Systems Store.

To place your order and claim your discount, go to

www.PureBodySystems.com

and enter your discount code

OUTSMART

CHAPTER 26

GET SCREENED FOR CANCER

Get regular screenings for common cancers and those that run in your family. We cannot screen for all cancers. Talk to your doctor about routine screening for breast, cervix, uterus, and ovarian exams (for women) and prostate exams (for men).

Everyone over 50, and depending on our personal or family history, earlier in life, should get routine colonoscopy and skin examinations. You and your doctor should decide at what age to start screening and the schedule and frequency of screenings for early detection.

Cervical Cancer

We live in an age where no woman should ever receive a cervical cancer diagnosis. With modern knowledge, proper screening, and attention to health and prevention, every women should have health. Get a complete women's health exam every year, including a breast

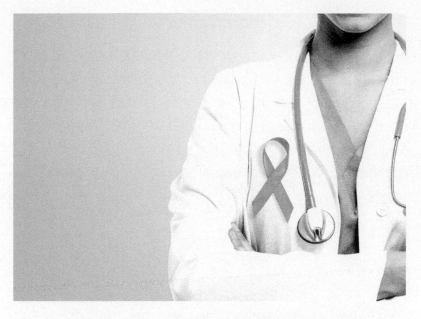

exam, pelvic exam of your reproductive organs, and PAP smear to screen for cervical cancer.

You may be at high risk for cervical cancer if:

You smoke, have used birth control pills for more than 5 years, have multiple births, do not practice safe sex, have multiple partners, have HIV, or take medications that suppress your immune system (lowering your capacity to fight infection).

You were born between 1940-1971 and your mother was given a hormone called DES during her pregnancy to prevent miscarriage. "DES Daughters" have a high rate of cervical cancer and should be screened for cervical cancer regularly.

Colon Cancer

Colon cancer is considered PREVENTABLE. Colon cancer is linked to dietary habits and food choices. Regular consumption of red meat and grilled foods have been linked to colon cancer. If you get regular screenings (colonoscopy), your doctor may find early rather than advanced changes at precancerous or early stages of cancer.

Discuss with your doctor.

Breast Cancer

Breast cancer screening should be individualized depending on breast density and individual and family risks and history. High breast density is a stronger risk factor for breast cancer than having a mother or a sister with breast cancer. Women with dense breasts get more breast cancers that are hard to detect on a routine mammogram.

All women should know their breast density so they can choose the right breast cancer screening approach. Get educated. Discuss with your doctor.

Don't gamble with your life!

Make health screening a part of your yearly health planning.

PART 3

Cultivate a Supportive Network of Family and Friends

CHAPTER 27

AVOID ISOLATION BY CULTIVATING NOURISHING RELATIONSHIPS

As life unfolds and the challenges of aging and illness arise, having a support system of family and nourishing friendships is vital.

Statistics show that cancer patients who have family support, a network of friends, community and support groups have better outcomes and better quality of life.

Isolation and loneliness are risk factors for cancer. People with good support systems live healthier longer lives and recover more successfully from illness.

Here are some ideas for giving yourself more support:

- Make an effort to **cultivate family, personal, and community relationships** that are nourishing and uplifting.

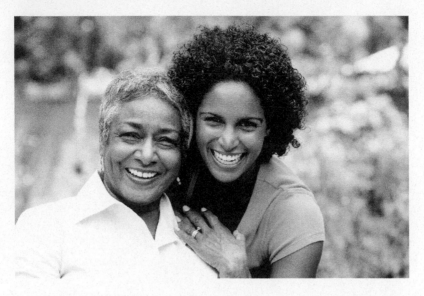

- Consider joining a club or local group that focuses on one of your hobbies or interests, and discover all the new friendships you can make. Reach out to an old friend or colleague purely for the joy of having a conversation with them.

- **Detox your relationships.** If a relationship is toxic or destructive, you can change your response and behavior to it, try to heal it – and if it cannot be healed (due to mental illness or abuse), then you can choose to separate from the toxicity of that connection.

- **Increase your oxytocin** (the brain chemical also known as the "trust or bonding hormone") by hugging someone every day.

You may be interested in www.mylifeline.org, a nonprofit organization that provides free personal websites to cancer patients and caregivers so they can easily connect with family and friends. The website's mission is to empower patients to build an online support community of family and friends to foster connection, inspiration, and healing.

No cancer patient or survivor should ever feel alone.

"Cancer is not a death sentence, but rather it is a life sentence; it pushes one to live."

Marcia Smith

CHAPTER 28

EXPRESS GRATITUDE AND APPRECIATION EVERY DAY

To enhance the quality of your life and the lives of those around you, express gratitude and appreciation every day. Count your blessings.

Acts of kindness, appreciation and thoughtfulness not only have a positive impact on your health and well being, but they also impact your friends and family, your community, and the larger world around you.

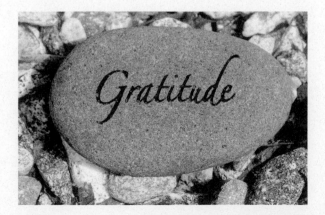

Cancer patients and cancer survivors benefit greatly from **cultivating habits of happiness**, which foster a robust immune response, less anxiety, improved capacity to cope with stress, change and loss, as well as greater optimism.

Here are tips from the Greater Good Science Center, seeds that can be planted and nourished in your life to cultivate inner peace and contentment, as well as robust immunity and resilience.

Habits of Happiness

1. Practice Gratitude. Take the time each day, perhaps at the dinner table with your family or at the end of your day in a journal, and share or write down 3 things that happened in your life today for which you are grateful. * These can be simple: a perfectly ripe peach, a profound realization that "My scan came back with no evidence of cancer," an acknowledgment that "I got to spend time with my son," or a declaration that "I woke up feeling really rested."

2. Write 3 lines at the end of each day that capture the essence of the day. What moved you? Made you laugh? Surprised you? (Make it a poem if you wish!)

3. Remember the sacred. Create a personal ritual in which you remember that you are part of something larger than yourself, whether you call that Nature, the Great Spirit, or God. This may be a moment of silence and prayer, lighting a candle, or remembering a time in your life in which you felt deeply connected. By doing this, you are "tending to the spirit."

4. Breathing exercise. Close your eyes. Settle down and relax in a comfortable position. Inhale softly, breathing in love and ease and a sense of well-being. Exhale softly and slowly, releasing your tension and stress. Allow yourself to just soften and open, relaxing on the breath.

"A happy person is not a person in a certain set of circumstances, but rather a person with a certain set of attitudes."

Hugh Downs

CHAPTER 29

LET OTHERS KNOW YOU CARE, AND THAT THEIR LOVE AND PRESENCE MAKES A DIFFERENCE

One of the most beneficial things you can do for your immune system is be kind to someone every day. Thoughtful words, gestures, and good deeds can help the people around you know that you appreciate them.

The same goes for being kind towards yourself.

Here is a powerful quote from Wayne Dyer, who summarizes the health-enhancing effect of kindness:

"The positive effect of kindness on the immune system and on the increased production of serotonin in the brain has been proven in research studies. **Serotonin** is a naturally occurring substance in the body that makes us feel more comfortable, peaceful, and even blissful. In fact the role of most anti-depressants is to stimulate the serotonin production to alleviate depression. Research has shown that a **simple act of kindness** directed toward another improves the functioning of the immune system and stimulates production of serotonin in both the recipient of the kindness and the person extending the kindness. Even more amazing is that persons observing the act of kindness have similar beneficial results. Imagine this: kindness extended, received, or observed beneficially impacts the physical health and feelings of everyone involved."

Wayne Dyer

Bottom line? Kindness is good for your immune system. So be kind to everyone you encounter, including yourself.

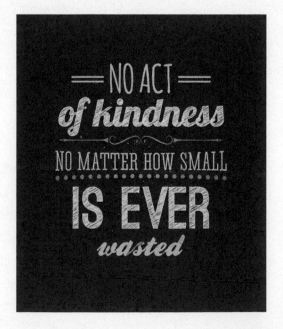

PART 4

*Include Extra Support and Protection
from Nutritional Supplements and
Herbal Medicines*

CHAPTER 30

TAKE 5 ESSENTIAL CORE NUTRITIONAL SUPPLEMENTS DAILY

Up to seven times as many **cancer patients survive and live more years*** when conventional treatment is combined with and followed by long-term use of herbal medicine and vitamins.

(Check with your health care provider before starting any new dietary or supplement program)

I recommend you take the following core supplements daily:

- **Multi vitamin/mineral** (copper-free and iron-free) to provide all of the essential micronutrients every day

- **Omega 3 Fatty Acids EPA and DHA Fish oils,** which are critical to normal immunity and normal inflammation, and which support a balanced mood

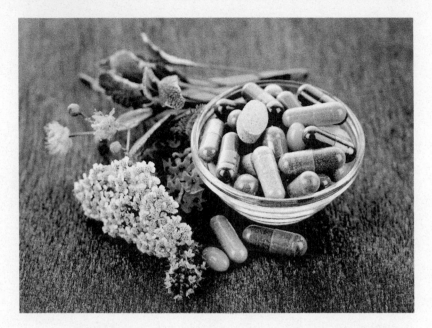

and healthy cell function. Vegetarians can opt for Organic High Lignan Flax Seed Oil as a source of fatty acids.

- **Vitamin D,** which normalizes cell-to-cell communication, impacts uncontrolled cell growth, and allows cells to differentiate into normal cells with a normal life cycle. Low levels of Vitamin D are associated with increased incidence of many cancers.

- **Probiotics/Acidophilus** to support the healthy friendly bacteria that are a crucial part of normal immunity, normal detoxification, and inflammation management. You can also get healthy friendly bacteria when you eat fermented foods such as yoghurt, miso, sauerkraut or kim chi.

- **Protein supplements** such as non heat treated,

undenatured whey protein or dairy free pea protein which are great for use in shakes and smoothies. I recommend 60-80 grams of protein daily (20 grams of protein = 3-4 oz serving). Other protein sources include but are not limited to beans and legumes, tofu, fish, chicken or poultry, high omega 3 eggs, grass-fed beef, lamb, or bison, Greek yoghurt, cottage cheese and almond butter.

- For both women and men: **Minerals**, including **Calcium and Magnesium** for bone support and normal cell function

- Consider using vegetable and fruit concentrates such as **green powders** from vegetable concentrates and **red powders** from fruit concentrates for extra cell-protective plant chemicals and antioxidants. This is also a great insurance policy if you do not eat 8-12 servings of fruits and vegetables daily, although you won't get the fiber, you will get lots of cell protective phytochemicals in the powders.

Taking these core supplements and important nutrients is a great way to strengthen your body's natural disease-fighting and cell protective capabilities.

* Learn More About How Cancer Survivors Live Longer with Herbal Medicine:

http://www.integrativecanceranswers.com/cancer-survivors-live-longer-with-herbal-medicine-and-vitamins/

CHAPTER 31

USE HERBAL ADAPTOGENS TO MODULATE THE EFFECTS OF STRESS AND SUPPORT A ROBUST IMMUNE SYSTEM

Adaptogens may be thought of as nourishing, replenishing and restorative plants, much like concentrated food. Typically, tonic adaptogen herbs enhance endurance and stamina and your ability to cope with and recover from stress.

Tonifying adaptogen herbs are considered to be more like concentrated foods...deeply nourishing and generally safe for long-term use (of course, always check with your health care provider before taking any herbal adaptogens or tonics).

Examples of Adaptogen Tonifying Nourishing Herbs include:

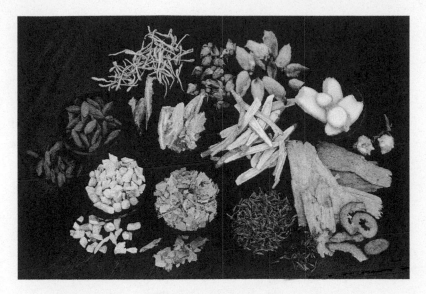

- **Astragalus** – a traditional Chinese herb that supports normal immunity.

- **Cordyceps** – a fungus that has been historically used for over 2,000 years throughout China and Asia as part of traditional nourishing tonics for a variety of conditions, including many cancers.

- **Rhodiola** – used by Russian Olympic athletes to promote stamina and endurance and modulate stress.

- **Siberian Ginseng** – a balanced tonic for supporting energy.

- **Red Ginseng** – an ancient plant traditionally used to support the ability to cope with stress, while supporting robust health and nourishing longevity.

- **Ashwagandha** – a traditional herbal medicine that has been used in India for hundreds of years for relieving fatigue and exhaustion associated with physical and emotional stress. It is appropriate for the person who feels "tired and wired," who is deeply exhausted but cannot relax.

- **Ganoderma Mushroom** – one of the great Asian "medicinal mushrooms" supporting normal immunity and inflammation function. Ganoderma has been used to relieve fatigue.

- **Shitake Mushroom** – another "medicinal mushroom" that is also an edible and tasty addition to vegetable dishes and soups.

- **Schizandra Berry** – the Chinese "Fruit of Five Flavors" used traditionally for balance and nourishment, rich in plant antioxidants.

- **Lycium Goji Berry** – a dried berry rich in antioxidants and cell protective nutrients, historically used for longevity.

- **Maca** – a South American plant rich in nourishing nutrients, traditionally used to support "recovery" from stress and illness.

Goji berry, Schizandra berry, and Sea Buckthorn Fruit are particularly interesting medicinal fruits that are considered to be among the "Imperial Herbs." They are plant medicines of extraordinary efficacy and extremely safe for long-term use. These three berries are also considered to be **Phyto (plant) Adaptogens** – plants that support the body in adapting to stress. Many Olympic athletes and high altitude climbers use these herbs to increase endurance and quench the free radicals and high levels of oxidative stress produced by strenuous activities and in extreme environments.

In addition, Rhodiola and Siberian (Eleutherococcus) Ginseng Herbal teas and extracts have been used by Olympic athletes to support stamina and endurance during the stress of training and high performance competition. (That can include the capacity to adapt to stress and the high performance demands involved in being a mom, a CEO, or a cancer patient!)

Under the supervision of a knowledgeable health care professional, herbal adaptogens, and the tonifying Imperial Herbs may be used effectively to find support health in the face of cancer treatment side effects, the stress of all phases of the cancer journey and to maintain and restore robust and vibrant healthy function.

"I can choose peace rather than this."

A Course in Miracles

Chapter 32

Work with an Integrative Health Practitioner Who is Focused on Health Rather than Disease

Choose a Wellness Doctor to Live Longer, Enhance the Quality of Your Life.

You may even find that as the years go by you may even save money as health is generally less costly than illness and a far better investment over the arc of time.

Patients and Functional Integrative health care providers observe that health focused **complementary and functional medicine** can yield lower lifetime costs, enhanced quality of life and sometimes more years of life and may even experience less overall suffering. Supporting health and healthy function makes a difference. You need both disease experts as well as health experts on your team.

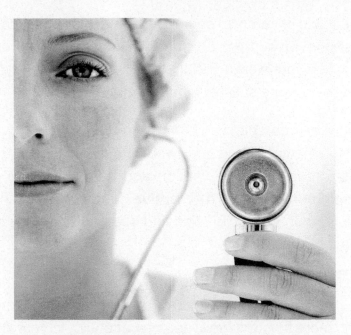

Complementary medicine, functional medicine, and integrative health care are all terms that refer to a holistic approach to health care – one that relies on your diet, nutrition, and healthy lifestyle habits, a consideration of you as a whole person, body, mind, emotions, and spirit as essential factors forming a strong foundation of health and wellness and your defense against illness. We believe in a team approach, integrating the best of all systems of medicine and healing, using the best tools from each arena and individualizing your health decisions for the best long term results and your highest quality of life.

Our current system is focused primarily on illness. We have a "disease care" system, not a health care system that is too often controlled or constrained by drug companies and insurance companies and managed care limitations. If you think outside the box of disease care and widen your view to include health focused care, you will enjoy a more satisfying outcome.

A recently published study on 150,000 patients over a 4-year period shows that when your doctor is interested in health and prevention and has knowledge of **Complementary and Alternative Medicine**, patients live longer and healthier lives and spend less money on health care!

Start looking for doctors who know about health and are interested in wellness. Look for doctors who choose to spend more time with you, and pay attention to your lifestyle factors such as diet, nutrition, exercise and stress. They may tend to prescribe fewer drugs and turn to complementary methods of promoting your health and healing. They teach you how to cultivate and sustain your vitality and health, rather than only chasing after symptoms.

Being under the care of a physician who is interested in you as a unique individual and in what causes health may save you money and extend your lifespan. Not to mention, you'll have improved quality of life!

If you want to have a voice in the direction of health care, take the time to write to your state and federal representatives and to your insurance companies. Talk to your employers who provide your insurance plans.

Ask for coverage for acupuncture, nutrition, herbal medicine, exercise, stress management, chiropractic, naturopathic care, homeopathy, yoga, stress reduction and meditation training. Many insurance policies today do cover acupuncture, chiropractic and nutritonal and lifestyle counseling on a limited basis.

Most changes in health care are consumer-driven.

Make your voice heard!

BONUS RESOURCE

*Organic Frozen Doctor-Nutritionist
Designed Meals*

Artisan Bistro Meals

If you are tired of the effort, energy, and expense it takes to shop for and prepare healthy organic food, then you will love Artisan Bistro Pro. And it is delivered right to your door!

These special **Doctor-Nutritionist Professionally Designed Artisan Bistro Pro frozen meals** are not found in health food stores or grocery stores. This is a special line of low carbohydrate, low glycemic, gluten-free, dairy-free, soy-free, nut-free, sugar-free, high protein paleo meals with a large serving of vegetables made from mostly organic ingredients.

Just what the doctor ordered! Perfect for staying on your meal plan and sticking to dietary guidelines. Perfect for supporting normal weight and body composition. Perfect for burning fat and building muscle (along with your exercise program and good stress management of course!)

I am probably one of the only persons who has NEVER eaten from a fast food chain in my entire life. (really!) And I NEVER buy frozen food, even in the health food store. That said, Artisan Bistro Pro meals are a great choice if you are searching for a more convenient way to prepare wholesome organic meals and just do not have time to purchase and prepare healthy organic food every day.

These meals are great solutions when you might be tempted to skip a meal, eat fast food or junk food, have ice cream for dinner or eat standing at your refrigerator door!.

Wouldn't it be great to just heat up a healthy meal that you ordered online or by phone and was shipped directly to you and be sitting down to dinner in 10 minutes?

Some of my favorites include:

• Roasted Red Pepper Chicken

• Wild Alaskan Salmon with Pesto

• Chipotle Barbeque Chicken

• Wild Alaskan Salmon with Balsamic Glaze

Artisan Bistro

Home Direct

To order your Artisan Bistro Pro meals,

visit www.ArtisanBistroDirect.com and enter your

Your Special Access Code 891418

Disclosure: We may receive commissions for some of the products mentioned. Trust us, we absolutely do not recommend anything we do not use ourselves. We recommend products that we simply love for all the right reasons.

"Life is not measured by the breaths we take, but rather by the moments that take our breath away."

Inspirational Cancer Quotes

Special Offer
from Dr. Nalini

Our Gift To You.

Get **10% Off Your First Order** for

Superior Professional Grade Supplements at our

Pure Body Systems Store.

To place your order and claim your discount, go to

www.PureBodySystems.com

and enter your discount code

OUTSMART

CREATE A BODY IN WHICH CANCER CANNOT THRIVE!

Dr. Nalini's

OUTSMART CANCER QUICK START GUIDE

**Enjoy Peace of Mind I Feel Confident I
Reduce Your Stress
Take Control of your Health and Your Destiny**

CREATE A BODY IN WHICH
CANCER CANNOT THRIVE

OUTSMART CANCER QUICK START GUIDE

GET ANSWERS TO YOUR
MOST COMMON AND MOST
PRESSING QUESTIONS

WHAT SHOULD I EAT?

WHICH SUPPLEMENTS SHOULD I TAKE?

Included in Your QUICK START GUIDE

Cancer Fighting Foods Recipes, Meal Plans
Which Foods to Eat
Which Foods To Avoid

The Most Important Immune Enhancing Protective
Nutritional and Herbal Supplements

How to Make Nutritious Delicious Fortifying Protein
Super Shakes

Turn on your cancer fighting genes
Choose nourishing protective anti-cancer super foods
Lose Fat Build Muscle
Control inflammation
Promote Healing and Repair

Optimize Nutrition Immunity and Energy
Protect your cells from damage
Promote longevity and vitality

**You are Invited to Join the
Integrative Cancer Answers Community**

Now that you've read the 32 Ways to OutSmart

Cancer, it's time to take the next step!

Get your

OUTSMART CANCER
QUICK START GUIDE

*Get Answers to
The Two Most Common and Most
Pressing Questions*

Go deeper into the material you've just learned.

Get instant access now!

www.integrativecanceranswers.com/outsmart-

cancer-quickstart-guide

Coming Soon:

Comprehensive Outsmart Cancer Plan which walks you step-by-step through each of the 32 Steps in this guide and shows you exactly what to do and MORE!

Complete with meal plans, recipes, and recommended supplements as well as lifestyle solutions, our programs are your next step to creating an anti-cancer body.

For more inspiration, tips and resources for creating vibrant health and longevity, visit:

www.IntegrativeCancerAnswers.com

ABOUT DR. NALINI CHILKOV

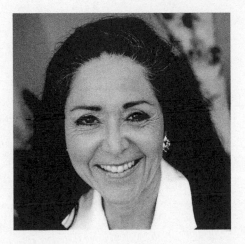

Dr. Nalini Chilkov, L.Ac., O.M.D. is a leading edge authority in the field of Integrative Cancer Care, Cancer Prevention and Immune Enhancement.

She is the Founder of IntegrativeCancerAnswers.com where she offers online programs and resources that empower and transform. Dr. Chilkov brings over 30 years of clinical experience combining the best of Modern Functional Medicine with the ancient wisdom of Traditional Oriental and Natural Healing. She is a highly respected expert in her field serving an exclusive celebrity clientele, a frequent speaker at conferences, educational institutions and a trusted resource to the media.

About Integrative Cancer Answers

We believe that cancer is a preventable disease.

We believe that every cancer patient deserves to live a vital life well beyond cancer.

If you are living with the stress, overwhelm and anxiety of cancer, suffering from the effects of difficult treatments, worried about cancer returning in the future or about getting cancer in the first place, Integrative Cancer Answers is designed for you.

We are committed to clearing up the confusion and providing you with safe, natural, easy to implement science based resources that will allow you to outsmart cancer, take control of your health and enjoy real peace of mind confident that you have access to the same time tested programs Dr. Chilkov has used for 30 years with thousands of people just like you to **get well, stay well and enjoy a long, vibrant and healthy life.**

Our answers give you confidence and peace of mind when pondering your most pressing health questions about cancer and making important life and health care decisions and choices.

Integrative Cancer Answers, founded by Dr. Nalini Chilkov, L.Ac., O.M.D. is committed to showing you **how to create a body and an environment in which cancer cannot thrive.** Our approach is informed by the best and most current modern science and research and functional complementary medicine and rooted in the wisdom of natural healing traditions and the fundamentals of vibrant health and robust immunity.

If you're looking for answers about what to do next, you've landed in the right place.

Our signature **Outsmart Cancer Programs** are the "at home" version of over 30 years of Dr. Nalini's experience and success in supporting people just like you through the cancer journey from diagnosis and treatment through restoration, recovery and life beyond cancer.

Our programs work with your body's own inherent natural healing mechanisms to promote your capacity to fight and become resistant to cancer and avoid getting cancer in the future or in the first place.

You Can Count on Integrative Cancer Answers:

- To **create a new framework** for healthy living, wholeness, and longevity

- To **create a holistic healthy environment** that

nourishes and promotes your body's own healing resources, enhancing your capacity to become
resistant to cancer

- To **tend to the whole person** inclusive of body,
mind, emotions and spirit

- To **be your #1 Trusted Source** for reliable information on Complementary Integrative Cancer Support

- To **foster a community of collaboration, caring
and support** in which all medical and healing systems join forces to find better solutions to outsmart
cancer

- To **Stay Abreast of Advances and Provide You
With Current, Up to Date Leading Edge Information** from around the world so that you can make
well informed choices with a feeling of confidence
and peace of mind

- To **Create Easy to Implement Step by Step Programs** so that you can thrive, feel vital and alive and
enjoy a superior quality of health and a long life

Our Mission is to empower people whose lives have
been touched by cancer to get well, stay well and live well
informed by science based, safe and natural solutions.

We want to teach you how to transform your body into
an environment inhospitable to the development, growth
and spread of cancer.

Visit the Community
Join the Conversation!

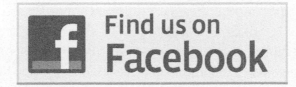

Join us today at

www.Facebook.com/DrNalini

For more resources and tips for

Outsmarting Cancer,

visit

www.IntegrativeCancerAnswers.com

INTEGRATIVE CANCER ANSWERS DISCLAIMER
and TERMS of USE

Our website, our products and programs DO NOT PROVIDE ANY MEDICAL ADVICE. It is the intent of Integrative Cancer Answers and Pure Body Systems LLC ("Company") to operate and offer products and programs consistent with the work of Dr. Nalini Chilkov, L.Ac, O.M.D. However, Company is not a health care practitioner or provider. Information provided on our websites, in this guide and in our products and programs is provided for informational purposes only and is not intended as a substitute for the advice provided by your physician or other health care professional or any information contained on or in any product label or packaging. You should not use the information on this web site or in or on any product label or packaging for diagnosing or treating a health problem or disease, or prescribing any medication or other treatment. You should always speak with your physician or other health care professional before taking any medication or nutritional, herbal or homeopathic supplement, or adopting any treatment for a health problem.

For any products or services purchased or downloaded from this web site, you should read carefully all product packaging and instructions. If you have or suspect that you have a medical problem, promptly contact your health care provider. Never disregard professional medical advice or delay in seeking professional advice because of something you have read on this web site. Information provided on this web site and the use of any products or services purchased from our web site by you DOES NOT create a doctor-patient relationship between you and any of the clinicians affiliated with our web site. Information and statements regarding dietary supplements have not been evaluated by the Food and Drug

Praise for Dr. Nalini

Dr. Chilkov is an invaluable resource for creating a plan for health in the midst of the challenges and complexities of cancer diagnosis, cancer treatment and recovery and investing in the health side of the equation.

Dr. Mark Hyman, M.D.
Five New York Times Best Sellers
UltraWellness, UltraMind, UltraMetabolism, The Blood Sugar Solution
Founder, The UltraWellness Center

Dr. Nalini Chilkov is my number one resource for cutting edge cancer info. She is on the leading edge of Integrative Cancer Care. I have sent my closest friends to her.

JJ Virgin, CNS, CHFS
Celebrity Nutrition and Fitness Expert
Best Selling Author, The Virgin Diet

When it comes to Integrative Cancer Care, Nalini Chilkov is my go to person.

Dr. Frank Lipman MD
Holistic Physician
Best Selling Author, Total Renewal

Dr. Chilkov's programs are masterful. You will feel empowered by her toolbox of natural medicines, as well as diet and lifestyle guidelines that are at the root of cancer prevention, cancer recovery and a long and healthy life.

Dr. Sara Gottfried, M.D.,
New York Times Best Selling Author The Hormone Cure

Made in the USA
Las Vegas, NV
15 August 2021

28222880R00090